200 Makeup Secrets: The Ultimate Guide to Flawless Beauty and Pro Tips

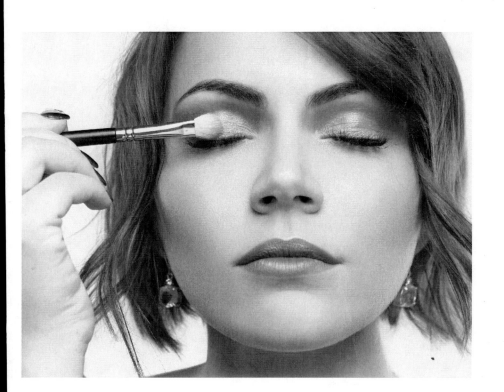

Contents of the book:

Introduction

Welcome to 200 Makeup Secrets: The Ultimate Guide to Flawless Beauty and Pro Tips! Whether you're a seasoned beauty lover or just beginning to explore the transformative world of makeup, this book is designed to be your go-to resource for mastering techniques, refining your skills, and discovering innovative hacks that will elevate your beauty routine.

In today's beauty landscape, makeup is about so much more than just products—it's a powerful tool for self-expression, creativity, and confidence. With these 200 curated secrets and pro tips, you'll gain insights that go beyond the basics. You'll uncover time-saving hacks, product-enhancing tricks, and subtle techniques that can completely transform your look. From prepping your skin for a flawless base to achieving the perfect smoky eye, these pages are packed with practical advice that can be easily adapted to suit any skill level, skin type, or desired look.

Each chapter dives into a different aspect of makeup artistry, breaking down techniques into accessible steps. You'll learn how to prep and prime your skin, master foundation application, sculpt with contour and highlight, enhance your eyes, and play with bold or natural lip looks. There's something for every occasion and style, whether you're aiming for a natural, glowing look or a dramatic, full-glam appearance.

Most importantly, this guide emphasizes that makeup is about embracing your unique beauty. We hope you feel inspired to experiment, try new looks, and find confidence in creating a makeup routine that's uniquely yours. So grab your brushes, your favorite products, and let's dive into the world of makeup secrets and pro tips that will have you looking and feeling your absolute best.

Skin Preparation

1.Moisturize Properly: Always start with a well-moisturized face. Use a moisturizer suited to your skin type—hydrated skin helps makeup apply evenly and look more natural.

2.Exfoliate Weekly: To achieve a smooth base, exfoliate your face once a week. This removes dead skin cells, allowing your foundation to glide on without emphasizing dry patches.

3.Use SPF Under Makeup: For daytime makeup, always apply SPF. Look for lightweight, oil-free sunscreens that won't interfere with your makeup. SPF powders can be great for touch-ups throughout the day.

4.Try a Hydrating Mist Before Primer: A quick spritz of a hydrating mist before applying primer adds extra moisture and helps prep the skin, especially if you have dry or combination skin.

5.Use a Primer Based on Skin Type: Primers are crucial for keeping makeup in place. For oily skin, use a mattifying primer; for dry skin, try a hydrating or illuminating primer.

Foundation and Concealer

6.Color Match in Natural Light: Always test foundation in natural light to find the right shade, as indoor lighting can alter how colors appear.

7.Apply Foundation with a Damp Sponge: Use a damp makeup sponge to apply foundation for a dewy, airbrushed finish that doesn't cake or look too heavy.

8.Layer Foundation Sparingly: Apply foundation in thin layers, building up only where needed. This technique prevents the "cakey" look and helps makeup stay natural.

9.Use a Color-Correcting Concealer: For dark circles, a peach or orange corrector cancels out blue undertones, while green can reduce redness.

10.Set with a Translucent Powder for Long Wear: To ensure foundation and concealer stay put, use a translucent powder to set them. This keeps makeup from slipping or creasing.

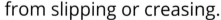

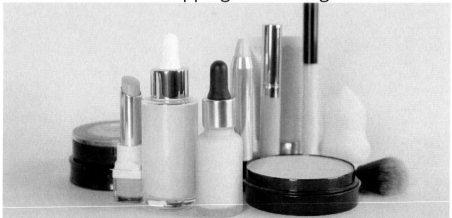

Blush, Bronzer, and Highlighter

11. Apply Bronzer in a '3' Shape: For natural-looking bronzing, sweep the bronzer in a "3" shape on each side of your face—from the forehead to the cheekbone and then the jawline.

12. Choose Blush Shades Based on Undertones: Pink tones suit cool undertones, while peach tones are flattering on warmer undertones. Experiment to find the most flattering hue for your skin.

13. Layer Cream and Powder Blush for Longevity: Apply a cream blush first, then set it with a matching powder blush. This technique creates a long-lasting, vibrant look.

14. Highlight High Points of the Face: For a natural glow, apply highlighter only to the high points—like the cheekbones, bridge of the nose, and brow bone.

15. Use Bronzer to Define the Eye Crease: Lightly dusting bronzer in your eye crease creates a cohesive look that subtly defines the eyes without needing extra eyeshadow.

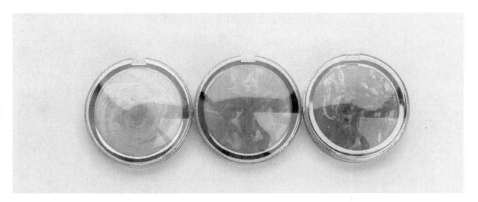

Eyeshadow Techniques

16.Prime Your Lids to Prevent Creasing: Eyeshadow primers are crucial, especially for oily lids. They create a smooth base and prevent shadow from creasing.

17.Start with Neutral Transition Shades: Using a neutral transition shade in the crease helps all your eyeshadow colors blend seamlessly and prevents harsh lines.

18.Layer Shadows from Light to Dark: For a gradient effect, start with a lighter base color, adding darker shades as you build up toward the outer corners or crease.

19.Use Setting Spray on Your Brush for Intensity: For metallic or shimmery shades, spritz your brush with setting spray before dipping into the shadow. This gives a foiled, high-impact look.

20.Blend, Blend, Blend: For a professional finish, use a fluffy blending brush to soften any edges. Blending creates a smooth transition between shades and prevents harsh lines.

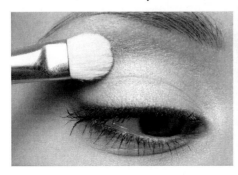 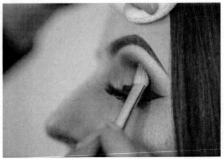

Eyeliner Tips

21.Tightline for Fuller-Looking Lashes: Use eyeliner on your upper waterline to create the illusion of fuller lashes. This technique is especially effective if you don't like visible eyeliner on your lids.

22.Use a Pencil for Smoky Looks: For a smoky eyeliner look, start with a pencil liner. Smudge it with a brush or cotton swab, then set it with a matching eyeshadow for lasting power.

23.Create a Guide for Your Wing: To create a symmetrical wing, start with a small dot or line at the end of each eye where you want the wing tip. Use this as a guide to ensure even wings.

24.Try Gel for Precision and Longevity: Gel eyeliners are great for precise lines and tend to last longer than pencils. Use an angled brush for best results.

25.Use Eyeshadow as Liner: For a softer look, use dark eyeshadow along your lash line. This adds definition without the harshness of traditional eyeliner.

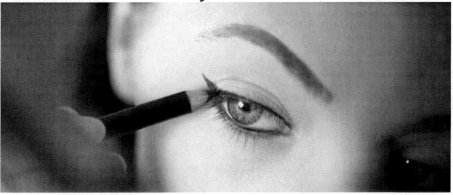

Eyelash and Mascara Tips

26. Curl Lashes Properly: Start curling at the base of your lashes, then gently "walk" the curler up to the tips. This creates a more natural, lifted look.

27. Heat Your Lash Curler for Extra Hold: Warm up your lash curler with a blow dryer (test it on your hand first!) before curling. The heat can make the curl last longer.

28. Use Mascara Primer for Extra Volume: A mascara primer coats your lashes, adding volume and length while helping the mascara stay longer and resist smudging.

29. Wiggle Mascara Brush at the Base: Wiggling the mascara wand at the base of your lashes before sweeping upward helps build volume and ensures every lash is coated.

30. Use Two Types of Mascara: For dramatic lashes, try layering two different formulas, such as a lengthening mascara first, followed by a volumizing one.

31. Use a Small Brush for Lower Lashes: A small or skinny mascara wand allows you to get close to the lower lashes without smudging or clumping.

32. Prevent Clumps by Wiping Wand: Before applying, gently wipe the mascara wand on a tissue to remove excess product. This helps avoid clumps and gives a cleaner application.

33.Apply Mascara to Both Sides of Lashes: For a fuller effect, apply mascara to both the tops and undersides of your upper lashes.

34.Use Clear Mascara for a Natural Look: For a minimal makeup day, clear mascara can define and hold your lashes without adding color, giving a naturally polished look.

35.Apply a Final Coat of Waterproof Mascara: If you're worried about smudging, finish with a coat of waterproof mascara to lock everything in place.

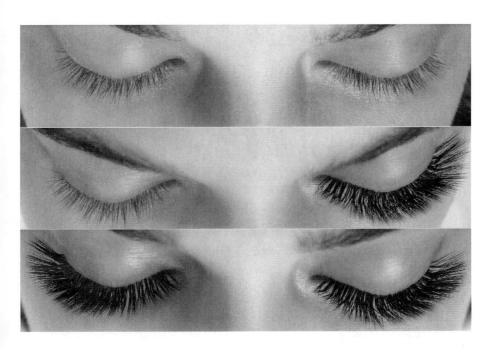

Eyebrow Shaping and Filling

36.Map Your Brows: For balanced brows, use the "rule of thirds": Align with the edge of your nostril for the inner edge, the outer nostril and pupil for the arch, and the outer nostril and outer corner of the eye for the end.

37.Use Short Strokes to Mimic Hair: When filling in brows, use short, hair-like strokes rather than one continuous line. This creates a natural, feathery look.

38.Comb Through After Filling: After filling in, use a spoolie to blend the product evenly through your brows, softening any harsh lines.

39.Highlight the Brow Bone: Apply a subtle highlighter or light shadow just below the arch of your brow to lift and define the brow shape.

40.Use Brow Gel for Hold: After filling in your brows, set them with a clear or tinted brow gel. This keeps them in place all day and gives them a polished look.

41.Match Your Brow Color to Your Roots: For the most natural look, choose a brow color that matches the roots of your hair.

42.Angle Brow Ends Slightly Downward: For a softer look, angle the tail end of your brows slightly downward rather than sharply horizontal or up.

43.Highlight Above the Brow Too: For extra definition, use a small amount of concealer or highlighter just above the brow to give them a lifted, clean look.

44.Brush Brows Upward: Brush brow hairs upward for a fuller, feathery look. This technique can also help you see sparse areas that need filling.

45.Keep Tweezing Minimal: Avoid over-plucking! Just clean up stray hairs beneath the brow and leave the natural shape as much as possible.

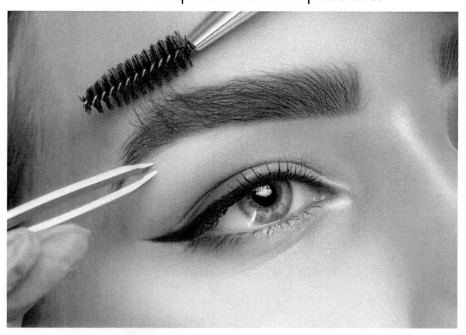

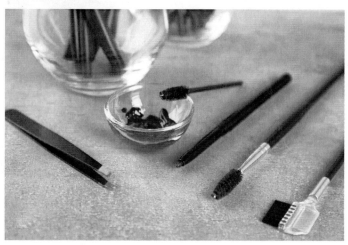

Lip Color and Application

46.Exfoliate Your Lips: Use a lip scrub or gently brush your lips with a toothbrush to remove dead skin, allowing lip products to apply smoothly.

47.Line Lips for Definition: Outline your lips with a lip liner to define their shape, prevent feathering, and extend the wear of your lipstick.

48.Overline Slightly for Fuller Lips: If you want fuller lips, slightly overline just above your natural lip line —especially on the top center and bottom center for a plump effect.

49.Apply Concealer Around Lips for Precision: After applying lipstick, use a small brush and a bit of concealer to clean up the edges for a super-defined look.

50.Layer for Long-Lasting Color: For a long-lasting lip, apply a layer of lipstick, blot with tissue, apply powder through tissue, and then add a final coat.

51.Use Lip Balm for Matte Lipsticks: Matte lipsticks can be drying, so prep your lips with a hydrating balm. Wait a few minutes before applying the lipstick.

52.Try Ombre Lips for Dimension: To create an ombre effect, apply a darker shade at the outer edges of your lips and a lighter shade in the center.

53.Use a Clear Gloss for a Plumping Effect: Apply a dab of clear gloss in the center of your lips to create a plumping effect, making lips look fuller.

54.Match Lip Liner and Lipstick: Choose a lip liner shade that's close to your lipstick color. This helps prevent harsh lines and makes the color look more natural.

55.Use Highlighter on Cupid's Bow: Add a touch of highlighter on the Cupid's bow (the center dip of your upper lip) to enhance your lip shape and add a glow.

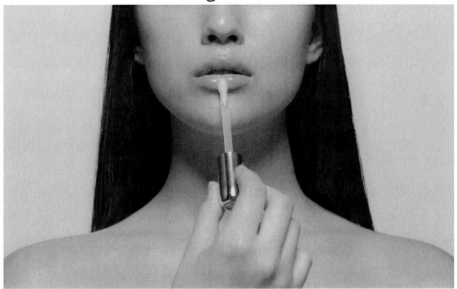

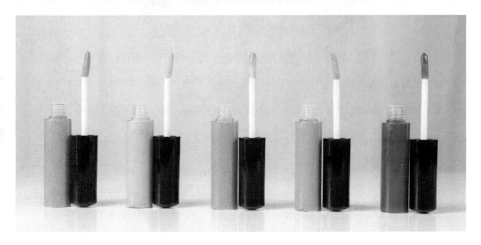

Contouring and Highlighting

56.Contour to Add Dimension: Use a contour shade in the hollows of your cheeks, along the jawline, and on the sides of your nose for added depth.

57.Use Cream Contour for a Natural Look: Cream contour products blend more naturally into the skin, providing a subtle, more skin-like finish.

58.Highlight Before Foundation: For a "lit from within" glow, apply highlighter before your foundation for a softer, more diffused effect.

59.Focus Highlighter on High Points: Apply highlighter only on the tops of the cheekbones, tip of the nose, and brow bone for a targeted glow.

60.Blend Contour Upward: When blending contour, always blend upwards rather than downwards to lift the face and avoid a muddy look.

61.Use a Beauty Blender for Cream Products: When working with cream contour or highlight, use a damp beauty blender to blend seamlessly without disturbing the base makeup.

62.Go Light on Nose Contour: For a natural nose contour, use a light hand and focus on creating soft, blended lines on either side of the nose.

63.Highlight Inner Eye Corners: Add a touch of highlighter to the inner corners of your eyes to brighten and open up the eye area.

64.Use Setting Spray for Dewy Highlight: For an

extra glow, spritz setting spray on your face after applying highlighter to help it blend and look more natural.

65.Layer Powders for Extra Intensity: For a bolder highlight, apply a cream highlighter first and then layer a powder highlighter on top for extra intensity.

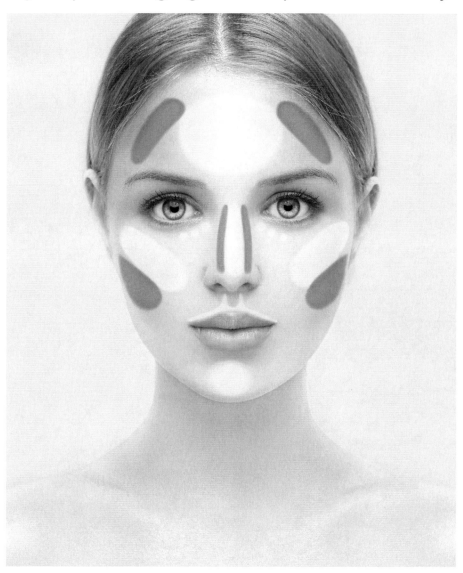

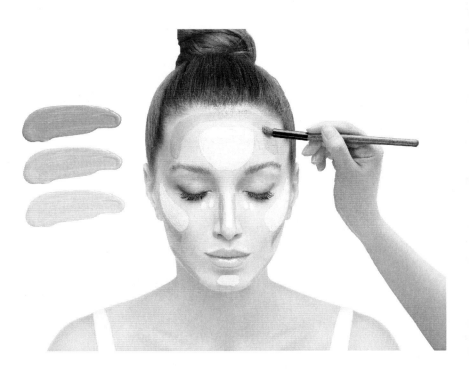

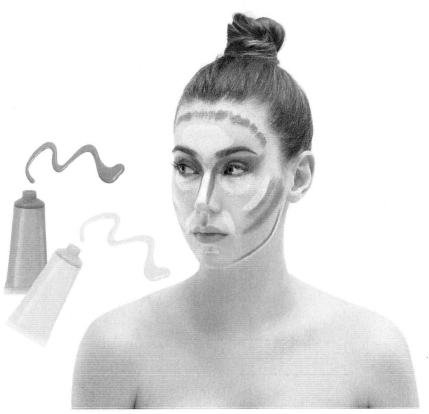

Makeup Setting and Longevity

66.Use Setting Spray as Final Step: Setting spray is the key to keeping your makeup locked in all day. It reduces powdery finishes and helps makeup melt into the skin.

67.Apply Setting Spray in Layers: Spritz setting spray after each major step (foundation, powder, eye makeup) to ensure every layer is set.

68.Use Powder Only Where Needed: Avoid over-powdering, which can make makeup look heavy. Instead, apply powder only in areas that tend to get oily, like the T-zone.

69.Touch-Up with Blotting Paper: For touch-ups, use blotting paper to absorb excess oil without disturbing makeup, then reapply a light dusting of powder if needed.

70.Use a Fan Brush for Powder: Use a fan brush for applying a light, controlled amount of powder to avoid a cakey finish.

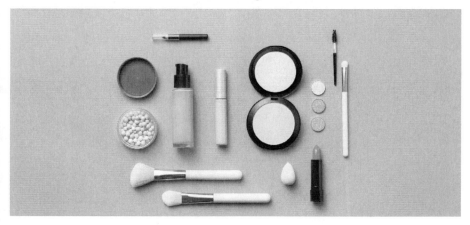

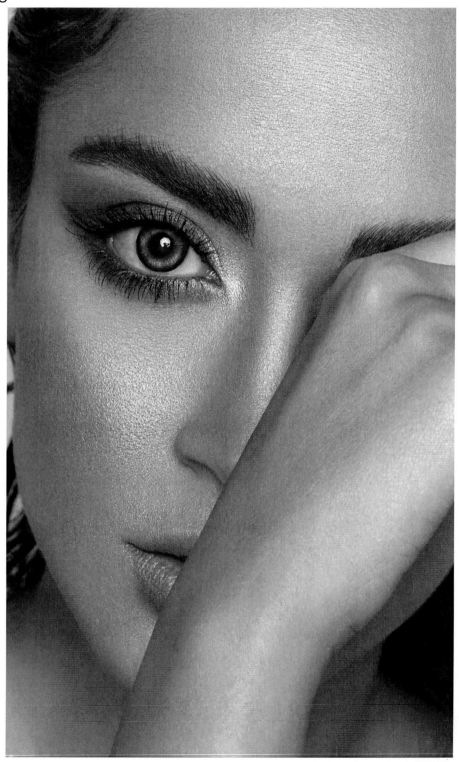

Advanced Skin Prep and Priming Techniques

71.Apply Ice to Depuff: If you wake up with a puffy face, gently rub an ice cube over your skin. This reduces swelling and tightens pores for a smoother canvas.

72.Use an Oil-Free Moisturizer for Oily Skin: If you have oily skin, opt for an oil-free moisturizer that hydrates without adding extra shine, making makeup adhere better.

73.Add a Glow with Illuminating Primer: For radiant skin, use an illuminating primer that contains light-reflecting particles. It enhances glow, especially under lightweight foundations.

74.Mix Primer with Foundation for Sheer Coverage: To create a more natural, sheer foundation, mix a small amount of primer with your foundation before applying.

75.Let Your Primer Set: Give your primer at least one minute to fully absorb before applying foundation. This ensures that the primer effectively grips the makeup.

76.Try Different Primers for Different Areas: If you have combination skin, use a mattifying primer in oily areas and a hydrating one on drier spots for a balanced base.

77.Use Eye Cream Before Concealer: Eye cream hydrates the under-eye area, preventing concealer from creasing or looking cakey.

78.Apply a Mattifying Balm After Foundation for Touch-Ups: For mid-day oiliness, lightly pat a mattifying balm on oily spots to absorb excess shine without disturbing makeup.

79.Create a Custom Primer with SPF: Mix a few drops of sunscreen with your primer for added sun protection, especially if your primer lacks SPF.

80.Use a Pore-Filling Primer Only Where Needed: Apply pore-filling primer on areas like the nose, forehead, and chin rather than all over to avoid a heavy feel.

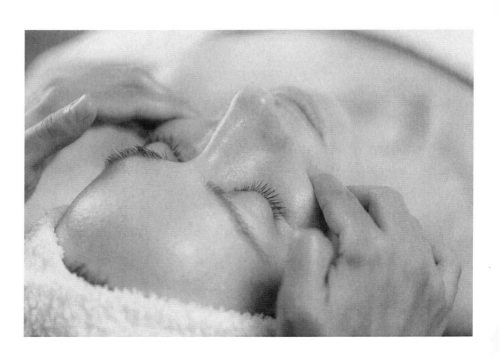

Perfecting Foundation Application

81.Dot Foundation Strategically: Place dots of foundation on the center of your face, then blend outward. This method ensures you get natural coverage where needed most.

82.Stipple, Don't Swipe: Use a stippling motion (small, tapping movements) to apply foundation with a brush or sponge. It helps avoid streaks and provides even coverage.

83.Warm Up Foundation on Your Hand: For cream or stick foundation, warm the product on the back of your hand before applying. This makes it more blendable.

84.Avoid Applying Foundation Directly Under Eyes: Skip applying foundation directly under the eyes to prevent a cakey look—use only concealer in this area.

85.Blend Foundation Down the Neck: Always blend foundation slightly down your neck to avoid a visible line between your face and neck.

86.Try Using Two Foundation Shades: Use a slightly lighter shade in the center of your face and a slightly darker shade around the edges to create natural dimension.

87.Set Foundation with a Pressed Powder for More Coverage: If you need more coverage, use a pressed powder with a powder puff instead of a loose powder.

88.Use a Kabuki Brush for Full Coverage: A dense, rounded kabuki brush helps to buff in foundation for full coverage without looking heavy.

89.Apply Foundation with Your Fingers for a Skin-Like Finish: For sheer coverage, use clean fingers to press foundation into the skin, mimicking the warmth and texture of your natural skin.

90.Revive Cakey Foundation with a Hydrating Mist: If foundation starts to look cakey, spritz a hydrating mist and pat lightly with a sponge to refresh the finish.

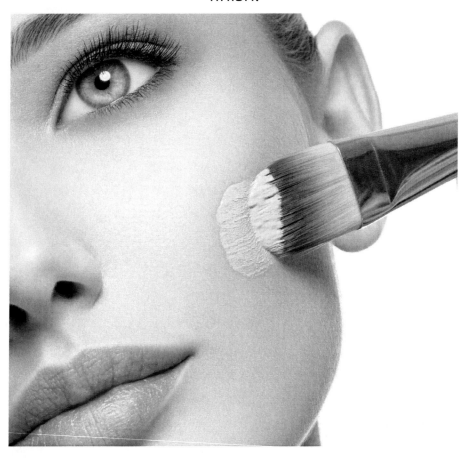

Concealer Tips for Flawless Coverage

91. Apply Concealer in a Triangle Shape: For under-eye brightening, apply concealer in an inverted triangle shape (under the eye and down toward the cheek) for a lifted look.

92. Use a Lighter Shade for Highlighting: Choose a concealer shade that's one or two shades lighter than your foundation to brighten under the eyes and high points.

93. Blend Concealer with Your Ring Finger: The ring finger has the gentlest touch, making it perfect for blending concealer under the eyes without tugging.

94. Let Concealer Sit for 1 Minute Before Blending: For more coverage, apply concealer, wait about a minute, then blend. It slightly thickens, giving more staying power.

95. Use an Orange Corrector for Dark Circles: For very dark under-eye circles, use a thin layer of an orange or peach corrector before applying concealer to neutralize blue tones.

96. Pat Concealer on Pimples, Don't Rub: When covering blemishes, pat concealer gently to build up coverage without disturbing the surrounding makeup.

97. Mix Concealer with Eye Cream for Hydration: If you have dry under-eyes, mix your concealer with a bit of eye cream. This keeps the area hydrated and prevents creasing.

98.Layer Thin Coats for Best Coverage: Rather than applying a thick layer of concealer, apply thin layers and build up gradually to avoid caking.

99.Brighten Shadows Around the Mouth: If you have shadowy areas around your mouth, apply a light layer of concealer to even out the tone.

100.Use a Powder Puff to Set Concealer: For crease-proof concealer, use a small powder puff to press setting powder under the eyes instead of brushing it on.

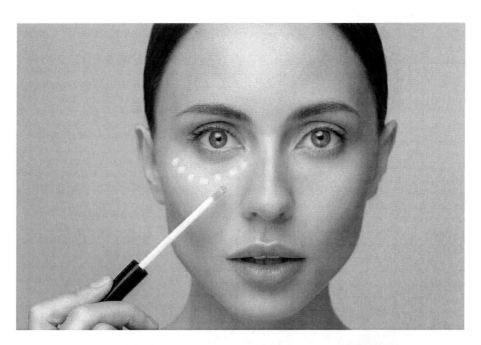

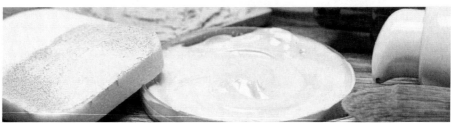

Expert Tips for Eyeshadow Blending and Application

101.Use a Transition Shade for Seamless Blending: Apply a neutral transition shade in your crease before darker colors to create a smooth gradient and avoid harsh lines.

102.Apply Shimmer with Your Finger: Shimmery eyeshadows often apply best with a finger, as it gives more pigment payoff and adheres better to the skin.

103.Use a Wet Brush for Metallic Shadows: For an intense, foiled look with metallic shadows, dampen your brush with setting spray before application.

104.Start with Eyes Before Face Makeup for Intense Looks: When creating bold eye looks, start with eyeshadow to avoid fallout on your foundation.

105.Choose the Right Brush for Blending: A fluffy, domed brush is best for blending shadows, while flat brushes work well for packing color on the lid.

106.Apply Concealer as Eyeshadow Primer: If you don't have an eyeshadow primer, a bit of concealer can help create a smooth base and even out any discoloration.

107.Pat, Don't Drag, Eyeshadow on the Lid: For better pigment, pat the eyeshadow onto your lid rather than dragging it, which can sheer out the color.

108.Highlight the Inner Corner for Bright Eyes: Apply a light, shimmery shade in the inner corners of your eyes to make them appear larger and more awake.

109.Try Layering Cream and Powder Shadows: For extra intensity, apply a cream shadow first and layer a powder shadow over it to set and deepen the color.

110.Use Tape for a Sharp Line: Place a small piece of tape along the outer corner of your eye before applying shadow to create a crisp, defined edge.

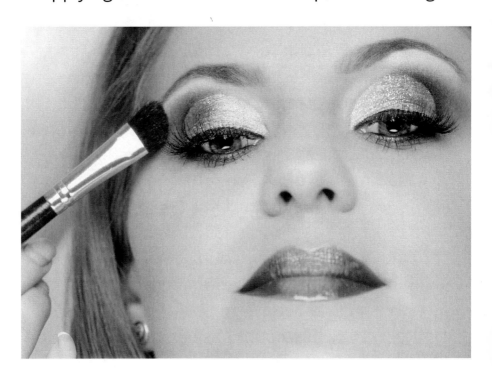

Advanced Eyeliner and Lash Tips

111.Use Eyeshadow as a Guide for Winged Liner: Create a soft wing with dark eyeshadow first; if you like the shape, go over it with eyeliner for a precise line.

112.Try White Eyeliner on the Waterline: Applying white or nude eyeliner on your lower waterline makes eyes appear larger and more awake.

113.Create a Smoky Liner with a Pencil: Draw a line with a pencil liner, then smudge it with a small brush for a soft, smoky effect.

114.Connect Top and Bottom Lines for Continuity: When lining both the upper and lower lash lines, connect them at the outer corner for a seamless, cohesive look.

115.Apply Mascara on Top of Falsies for Blending: If using false lashes, add a coat of mascara after applying them to blend your natural lashes with the falsies.

116.Trim False Lashes to Fit Your Eye Shape: If falsies are too long, trim them from the outer edge to fit your eye shape for a natural look.

117.Layer Eyeliner on Waterline for Extra Intensity: For dramatic eyes, apply eyeliner on the upper waterline to intensify the lash line without adding visible liner on the lid.

118.Use Tweezers for Precise Lash Application:
Apply false lashes with tweezers for better control,
especially when positioning close to the lash line.

119.Curl Lashes Before and After Mascara (Gently!):
Curl lashes before applying mascara, then give them
a gentle curl afterward for an even stronger lift.

120.Coat Both Sides of Lashes for Full Coverage: For
a bolder lash look, coat both the tops and bottoms
of your lashes with mascara.

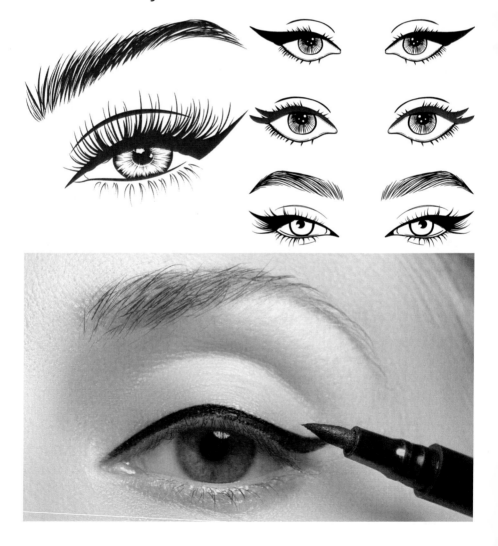

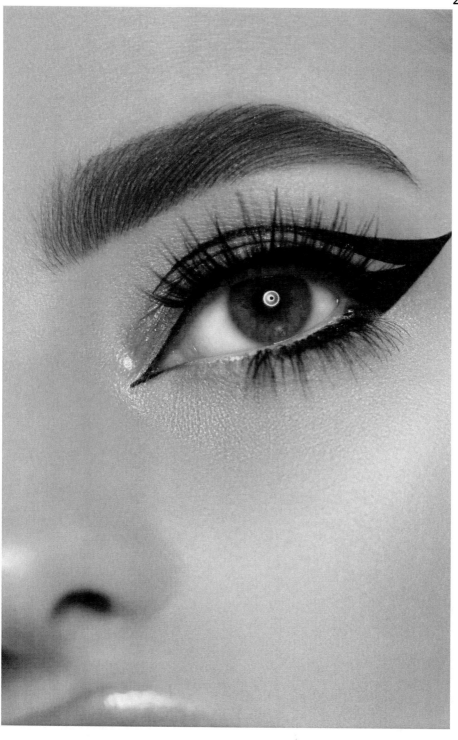

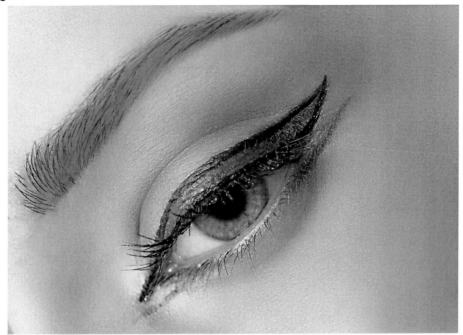

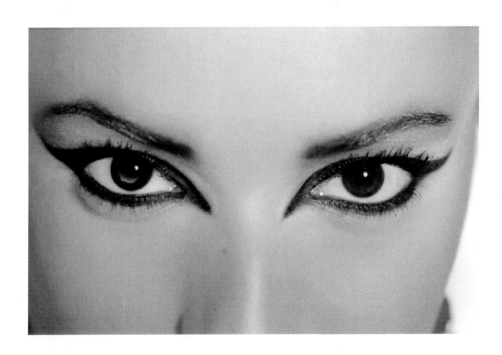

Unique Makeup Hacks and Tricks

121.Use Lip Balm as a Highlighter: If you're out of highlighter, dab a bit of clear lip balm on the high points of your face for a natural, dewy glow.

122.Turn Lipstick into Blush: Dab a little lipstick on your cheeks and blend with your fingers or sponge for a coordinated blush that matches your lip color.

123.Apply Concealer in an Upside-Down Triangle Under Eyes: An upside-down triangle shape brightens the entire under-eye area, not just under the lash line, giving a lifted effect.

124.Use Eyeshadow as Brow Powder: In a pinch, a matching eyeshadow shade can double as brow powder for filling in sparse brows.

125.Set Lipstick with Translucent Powder through Tissue: Apply a tissue over your lips after applying lipstick, then dust translucent powder over the tissue. This sets the lipstick without dulling the color.

126.Create a Smoky Eye with Just Eyeliner: Apply pencil eyeliner along your lash line, then use a smudger brush to blend it upward for an instant smoky effect.

127.Use a Business Card for Mascara Application: Place a business card behind your lashes to keep mascara from smudging on your eyelid, especially with lower lashes.

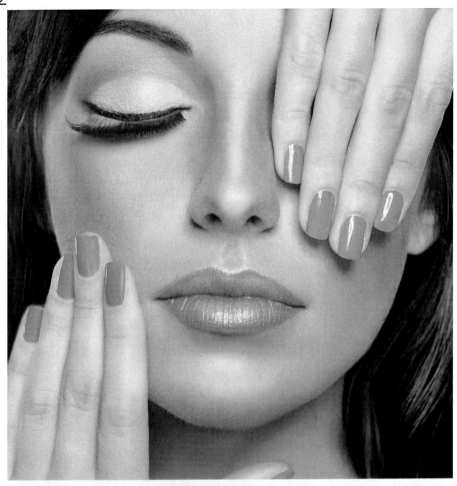

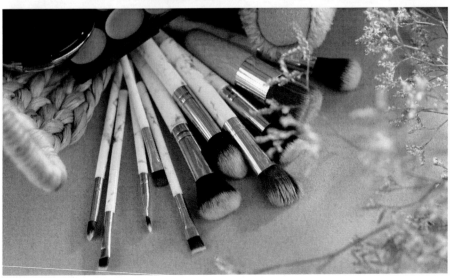

128.Apply Primer to Lashes Before Mascara: A thin layer of face primer on your lashes before mascara can add volume and help mascara stay on longer.

129.Contour Lips for a Fuller Look: Apply a slightly darker shade of lip liner around the edges of your lips and blend inward before applying lipstick to give your lips more dimension.

130.Mix Foundation with Facial Oil for Dewiness: For dry skin or a dewy look, mix a drop of facial oil with foundation for a radiant, hydrated finish.

131.Layer Blush for Long-Lasting Color: Use a cream blush first, then set it with a powder blush in a similar shade. This layering technique ensures blush lasts all day.

132.Use a Spoon to Create a Perfect Winged Liner: Place the handle of a spoon at the outer corner of your eye to create a straight line for your winged eyeliner, then use the rounded edge to perfect the curve.

133.DIY Tinted Moisturizer: Mix a bit of your foundation with moisturizer to create a lightweight, tinted moisturizer that's perfect for natural days.

134.Use Concealer to Define Brows: Apply concealer along the edges of your eyebrows and blend to make your brows look sharper and more defined.

135.Use Clear Lip Gloss for a Wet Eyeshadow Look: Apply a little clear lip gloss over any eyeshadow for a glossy, editorial look.

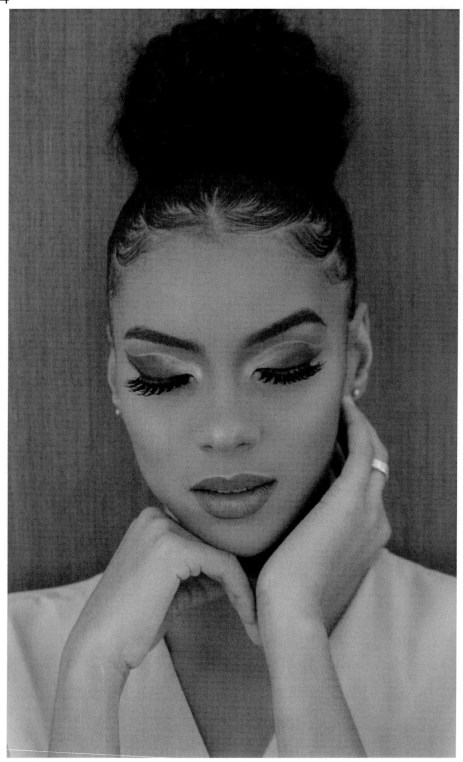

136.Repurpose Mascara as Liquid Liner: Use a thin brush dipped in your mascara wand to create eyeliner if you're out of liquid or gel liner.

137.Apply Foundation in Center of Face First: Start applying foundation in the center of your face (where most redness occurs) and blend outward for a natural look without heavy coverage around the edges.

138.Press and Roll Powder into Skin for a Flawless Finish: Instead of sweeping powder, press it into your skin with a puff or sponge. This technique sets makeup without moving it around.

139.Use Setting Spray Between Layers: Spritz setting spray after each layer (primer, foundation, powder) to "lock in" makeup and make it last much longer.

140.Fix Broken Powder with Rubbing Alcohol: If your powder makeup breaks, add a few drops of rubbing alcohol, press it back together, and let it dry. It'll be good as new!

141.DIY Lip Scrub with Sugar and Honey: Mix sugar and honey for a natural lip scrub. Exfoliating your lips regularly will make lipstick apply smoothly.

142.Apply Blush According to Face Shape: For round faces, apply blush along the cheekbones to elongate; for heart-shaped faces, apply on the apples of cheeks for balance.

143.Use Bronzer as an Eyeshadow: Bronzer can double as an eyeshadow for a monochromatic look that's natural and warm.

144.Apply Blush Over Nose Bridge for a Sun-Kissed Look: Lightly dust blush over the bridge of your nose to mimic a natural sun-kissed glow.

145.Heat Up Pencil Eyeliner for Smooth Application: Warm up your eyeliner pencil with a lighter (for just one second!) to make it glide on more smoothly and give a gel-like consistency.

146.Use Translucent Powder to Make Any Lipstick Matte: Dust a light layer of translucent powder over your lipstick with a tissue in between to mattify any lipstick.

147.Create a Contour Guide with a Spoon: Place a spoon under your cheekbone to easily see where to apply contour, giving you a natural, lifted look.

148.Use a Beauty Blender in Place of Blotting Paper: If you're shiny, dab a dry beauty blender on oily areas. It absorbs excess oil without removing makeup.

149.Use Eyeshadow to Enhance Lip Color: Add a dab of eyeshadow in the center of your lips to create a unique shade or an ombre effect.

150.Layer Lip Products for Dimensional Lips: Apply a darker lip liner, a base lip color, and a dab of lighter gloss in the center for a full, 3D effect.

151.Highlight Shoulders and Collarbone for Glow: For a radiant body glow, apply highlighter on your shoulders and collarbones, especially for special events.

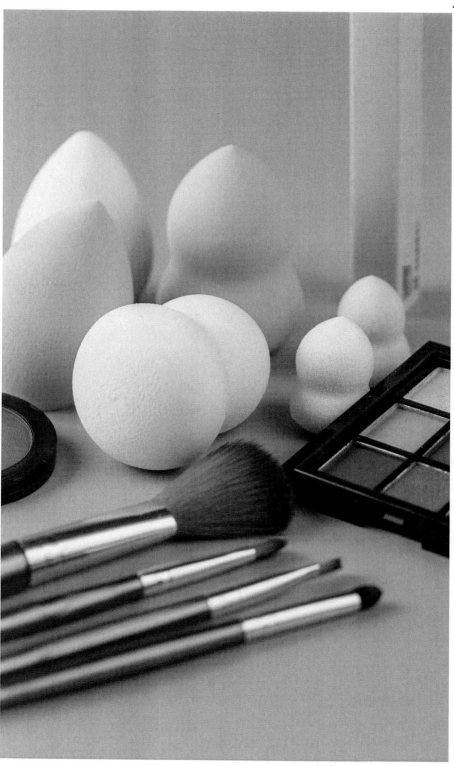

152.Make Your Own Brow Gel: If you're out of brow gel, spray hairspray on a spoolie and brush it through your brows for a similar effect.

153.Use Highlighter as Eyeshadow for a Cohesive Look: Apply your face highlighter on your eyelids as eyeshadow to create a coordinated, glowing look.

154.Mix Eyeshadow with Setting Spray for Liner: Dip a small liner brush in setting spray, then pick up eyeshadow to create a custom-colored eyeliner.

155.Use Cotton Swabs for Cleanup: Dampen a cotton swab with micellar water to easily clean up mistakes around eyeliner or lipstick.

156.DIY Brow Pomade with Old Mascara: Clean out an old mascara tube, add a bit of brow powder, and mix with a drop of oil for a makeshift brow pomade.

157.Create the Illusion of Fuller Lips with Concealer: Apply a small amount of concealer just above your Cupid's bow and below your bottom lip line, then blend.

158.Set Cream Products with Matching Powder Products: For long-lasting results, layer powder blush over cream blush, or powder bronzer over cream bronzer.

159.Use Lip Balm to Tame Flyaways: Smooth down flyaways with a little clear lip balm for a quick fix in a pinch.

160.Apply Eyeshadow with Your Finger for More Pigment: For bolder color, especially with shimmers, use your finger to press shadow onto your lid.

161.Use Ice Water to Set Makeup: Dunk your face in ice water for a few seconds after applying makeup (Japanese "Jamsu" technique) to set everything and achieve a matte finish.

162.Create Fake Freckles with Brow Pencil: Lightly dot a brow pencil across your nose and cheeks, then pat gently with your finger to soften for a natural freckle look.

163.Use Concealer as a Lip Primer: Apply a little concealer over your lips before lipstick to cancel out natural lip color and make the lipstick shade pop.

164.DIY Color-Correcting Primer: Mix a drop of red or green pigment with your primer to create custom color-correcting primers.

165.Place Bronzer on Outer Forehead: For a sunkissed effect, apply bronzer along the outer perimeter of your forehead and blend toward the hairline.

166.Use a Toothbrush to Exfoliate Lips: Gently brush your lips with a toothbrush to exfoliate and create a smooth base for lipstick.

167.Make Lashes Look Fuller with Tightlining: Apply eyeliner to your upper waterline to make lashes appear thicker without visible liner.

168.Use Light Powder to Brighten the Under-Eyes: After concealer, dust a brightening powder under your eyes to set and add extra brightness.

169.Turn Old Mascara Wand into a Brow Tool: Clean an old mascara wand and use it as a spoolie to brush and shape brows.

170.Outline Lips with Concealer for Clean Edges:
Use a small concealer brush to outline your lips after applying lipstick for a crisp, defined edge.

171.Make Eyeshadow Pop with White Eyeliner Base:
Apply white eyeliner on your lids before shadow to intensify the color and make it stand out.

172.Use Concealer to Correct Makeup Mistakes: Dab concealer around eyeliner or lipstick mistakes instead of wiping away everything for a quick fix.

173.DIY Glossy Eyelids with Vaseline: For a glossy lid look, dab a small amount of Vaseline on top of your eyeshadow (skip mascara to avoid smudging).

174.Contour with Two Shades for a Natural Look:
Use a lighter contour shade in the hollows of your cheeks and a slightly darker shade along the jawline for a more blended look.

175.Make Cream Blush with Lipstick: Swipe lipstick on the back of your hand and apply it to your cheeks as a cream blush for an easy, cohesive look.

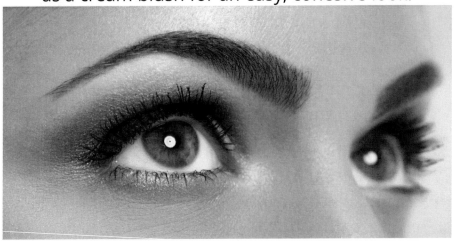

More Advanced and Creative Makeup Hacks

176.Make Eyes Appear Bigger with Two Mascaras: Apply a lengthening mascara on the upper lashes and a volumizing mascara on the lower lashes for a balanced, eye-opening effect.

177.Use Baby Powder for Lash Volume: Dust a bit of baby powder on your lashes between mascara coats for thicker, fuller lashes.

178.Create a Lip Tint with Powder Blush: Tap some powder blush onto your lips and finish with clear lip balm for a long-lasting, natural lip tint.

179.Apply Foundation on Ears for a Uniform Look: If you're wearing your hair up, apply a light layer of foundation on your ears to keep them from looking red compared to your face.

180.Warm Up Concealer for Better Blending: Rub a bit of concealer between your fingers to warm it up before applying—it helps with smoother blending.

181.Use a Small Blush Brush for Contouring: A smaller blush brush gives you more control when applying contour, especially in tighter areas like the nose.

182.Use Setting Spray on Brow Brush for Longevity: Spritz your brow brush with setting spray before applying brow powder to help it last all day.

183.Make Highlighter Pop with Setting Spray: Dampen your highlighter brush with setting spray before applying for an intense, glowing highlight.

184.Layer Gloss on Matte Lipstick for Dimensional Color: Apply a gloss only on the center of matte lipstick for a fuller, multi-dimensional effect.

185.Use Clear Lip Gloss as a Dewy Cheek Highlighter: For a natural, dewy highlight, dab a small amount of clear gloss onto your cheekbones.

186.Apply Highlighter on Collarbone and Shoulders: Sweep highlighter across your collarbones and shoulders for an overall glow that's great for evening events.

187.Use Nude Eyeliner on the Lower Waterline for Brighter Eyes: For a subtle brightening effect, use nude eyeliner on the lower waterline instead of white for a more natural look.

188.Create the Perfect Cupid's Bow with an 'X': Draw an 'X' on the Cupid's bow with lip liner, then outline and fill in the rest of your lips for a precise shape.

189.Add a Drop of Oil to Thick Concealers: If your concealer is too thick or drying, add a drop of facial oil to make it creamier and more blendable.

190.Brush Your Brows Upward for a Fluffy Look: Use a spoolie to brush your brows upward, giving them a fuller, feathery appearance that's on-trend.

191.Apply Blush Higher on the Cheeks for a Lifted Look: Placing blush higher on your cheekbones instead of the apples gives a more lifted, sculpted appearance.

192.Use Light Concealer on Inner Eye Corners to Brighten: Dab a small amount of light concealer on the inner corners of your eyes to create an awake and bright look.

193.Blend Foundation with Your Neck Shade: For a natural match, blend foundation to match your neck rather than your face to avoid stark color differences.

194.Use Vaseline for an All-Over Glossy Effect: Dab a tiny bit of Vaseline on your eyelids, cheeks, and lips for a cohesive, glossy, dewy look.

195.Use Eyeshadow as a Root Touch-Up: If you're in a pinch, apply eyeshadow that matches your hair color to cover up roots temporarily.

196.Cut Crease Guide with a Spoon: Use the rounded edge of a spoon as a guide for creating a perfect cut crease with your eyeshadow.

197.Use Red Lipstick to Neutralize Dark Circles: Apply a thin layer of red or peach lipstick under the eyes (especially on deep dark circles), then cover with concealer to brighten.

198.Powder Lips Before Lipstick for Longevity: Dust translucent powder over your lips before applying lipstick to help it adhere and last longer.

199.Outline Bottom Lip for Fuller Look: Draw a thin line of highlighter just under the center of your bottom lip for an illusion of fuller lips.

200.Apply Highlighter Over Setting Spray for Dewy Finish: Apply highlighter after misting your face with setting spray. It blends into the skin more naturally, giving a dewy, radiant look.

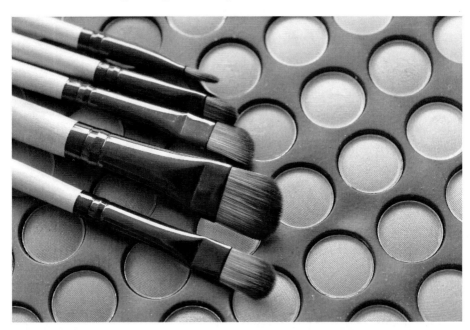

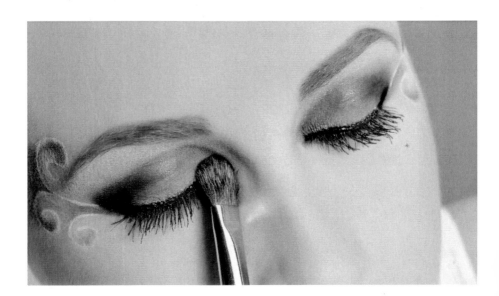

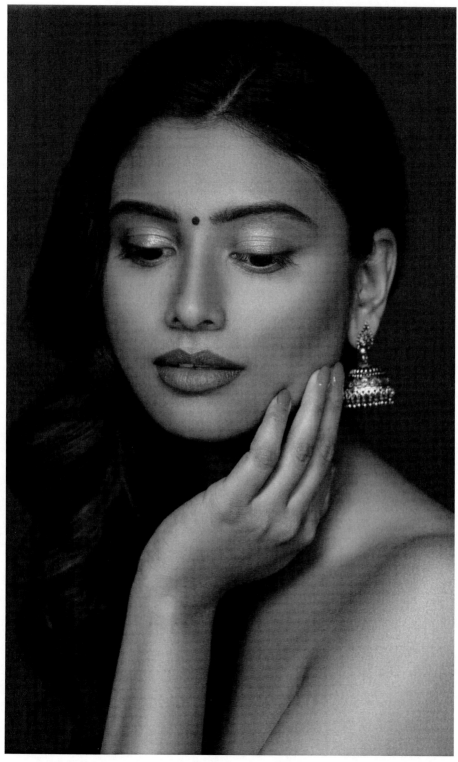

Conclusion: Embrace Your Unique Beauty, and Let Us Know Your Thoughts

Congratulations on reaching the end of 200 More Makeup Secrets! We hope this guide has sparked inspiration, boosted your confidence, and provided you with a treasure trove of techniques to keep your makeup routine fresh and exciting. As you experiment with these tips, remember that makeup is a journey, and every stroke of the brush or swipe of color is part of your creative expression.

No matter your skill level or style, these pages are meant to empower you to embrace your unique beauty, explore trends fearlessly, and make every look your own. The art of makeup is constantly evolving, and you are now part of that evolution, equipped with advanced techniques and insider tricks to confidently create, play, and perfect any look.

We'd love to hear from you! Your feedback helps us continue improving and innovating, and it's always inspiring to hear how these tips work for you. Did you find new favorites? Are there any other areas of makeup you'd love to explore in the future? Share your thoughts, ideas, and favorite discoveries with us. Leaving a review or sending your feedback is a small gesture that can make a big impact.

Thank you for being a part of this beauty journey—
your voice matters, and we can't wait to see where
your creativity takes you next!

Made in United States
North Haven, CT
16 June 2025

69849324R00030